Parkinson Disease

"Wind in the body"

About the Author

Shirley Lopez, I am the author who wrote this piece and I suffer from Parkinson Disease since 2012 as diagnosed by doctors, however I suspect that my problem began way before then but not diagnosed. Over the years I have lost the use of my legs had the shakes and suffered from Sun downing. I was over-weight, nervous wreck, and stressed beyond on belief. I decided to take control of my life and turn it around no doctor or family member could do this for me. It took my sheer will power and the grace of God. I prayed about this because I was tired of being in a wheel chair, a nervous wreck, over weight and just generally over all miserable.

At this point in my life everything was all wrong! I made up my own diet program none of these commercial deals. I knew good food and what I was chowing down on was horribly wrong for me. My legs were cramping me so bad I did not want to walk due to the fact I did not drink water but consumed too much caffeine. I cut down on Pepsi cola my weakness coffee gives off the same effect. I started drinking more water. I went upstairs to our exercise room and twice a day rode the bicycle first it was only five minutes then ten and finally half an hour 2X's each day. I had to take my right foot and push the pedal making the left side work in unison. It was painful at first but I did it because God was with me.

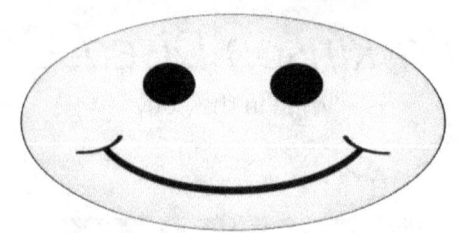

I finally went from210 pounds to 150 pounds from a size 1X to a normal size of 14. Lost enough weight that I could stop taking insulin. Yes, I had become a diabetic. I had a mild heart attack and other health problems. I realized my being overweight was causing me a lot of grief. I took my life in my hands! With the help of God, I turned myself around spiritually and physically. Now my friends say to me why are you so happy. They remember me when I was Ms. Gloom and Doom!

You only live life once so be **"Happy"** and live it with **Gusto!** Do you really like being sick? Not being able to enjoy your family and life in general. Yes, **God answers prayers** but unlike our natural parents he does not give it to us on **a "silver platter."** We are expected to work for what we receive not just put our hand out! He supplies our every need but not our wishes. We must be able to work for it. He expects us to do more than just ask. **Pray but then get off your duff and do something about it!**

This book was written as an informational piece not for medical advice. You should always consult your physician before you attempt to try any of my methods. Also, it is meant as an inspirational piece for those who truly do have faith in God. We all have an Angel who guides and protects daily. Those of you who believe in Angels will find comfort in this knowledge. My Angel is with me daily and during the night as well. It is not meant for us to walk alone. There is a physician who can cure everything with just the wave of his hand.

This great physician walked amongst us and helped us to understand that the heavenly father has prepared for us a place where we will not suffer any more the heart aches, pain, and suffering that binds us to this world. We must remember that when we are going through our trials. We will not always be able to overcome our weakness that our body has as we are slowly decaying. It is meant for us to take knowledge in the hope of our resurrection to a new body.

While we exist on earth we can take control of our lives even if we suffer from Parkinson Disease, family issues, financial problems, worldly events, and any other thing that affects us. First and foremost, it is not within us to prevail without the help of our heavenly father. It is no secret what God can do. You will never walk alone as no power can conquer you if you put God on your side. Just take God at his promise to you. It really is no secret his power and with arms wide open he will pardon you. Then he will stand by you and protect you.

Time only gives you the ability to make amends

Contents:

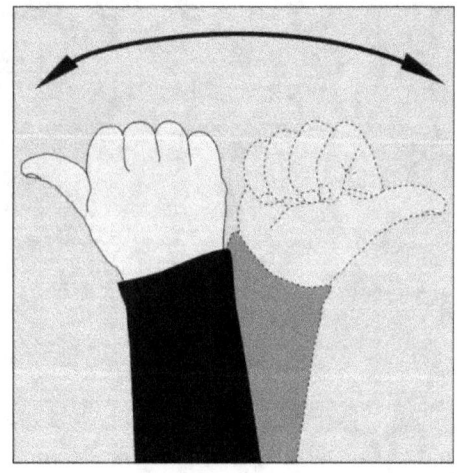

While Parkinson Disease effects different people in many ways there are some signals that will let a person know that they have the disease. These signals are what the Neurologist use when they are diagnosis of a patient.

1.) One of the first signs that is evident in most people is that of having tremors or a shaking. This usually begins in one of your limbs such as your hand or fingers.
2.) Next is slowed movement known as bradykinesia.
3.) Many people suffer with rigid muscles and often think that they have RA when in deed it is another symptom of Parkinson.
4.) The posture soon becomes impaired because of pain a person is not able to sit correctly and even may lean.
5.) The loss of automatic movements slows down tremendously. You find that your dropping things because you just can't get there in time.
6.) One of the worse things for me was when my speech began to change. I could not say my words correctly twisting them around.
7.) One of the last notable changes is the ability to write. Cursive becomes so bad it is not recognizable. As a professional writer

Being able to recognize the symptoms in yourself is very vital. You do not need to give in to those symptoms instead fight each one. We will talk about the ways you can fight those symptoms soon.

Also, there are five stages of Parkinson Disease and enable yourself to approach each stage at a slower pace. Many people live a long life. Some are happy and do many things.

Michael J Fox is a shining example of this but perhaps you know someone in your life who has the disease. Others unfortunately just fold up and give up. You can help us fight the disease by taking an interest and not being judgmental. Often a person with Parkinson Disease might be happy one day and doing a lot of things several days or the next day not able to hardly move. Even worse depression and sun downing haunts all Parkinson people.

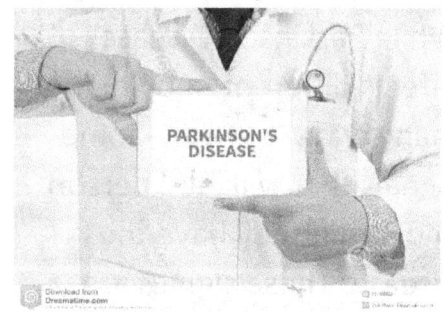

Take Time to Be Patient with US

One of the major things people have problems with is called sun downing. When it is time for the sun goes down we get up. I have gone as high as four days and nights without sleeping and that my friends greatly affect my ability to function.

I am happy jack all the time walking with a very fast pace or just hiding in the bedroom not want to get up and out. People tell me slow down. How can I slow down when my mind is racing and my body is trying to keep up? I run instead of walking! Everything is at a fast pace. Like right now I am typing so fast you would not believe it.

8

I listen to fast music to keep my mind going. I cannot sleep and am on the go. I want to drive my car fast, run, just go!

go! But tomorrow I will not want to move. My body will ache and I will be stiff. Odds I will get depressed and not talk to my friends at all. Keep myself locked up in my apartment.

Depression is another key problem that most Parkinson people suffer from time to time. There is no need to suffer over long periods of time because your doctor will give you medication that helps to combat depression. But this is not to be confused with bi-polar disorder. Those who suffer with bi-polar depression usually have mood swings that happen very quickly or can be seasonal. Parkinson people depression knows no season and it usually hits without relief unless you get a controlled medication.

Who coined the phrase Parkinson Disease?

The person who first coined the phrase Parkinson disease was a doctor out of England by the name of James Parkinson. In India, it is referred as *"wind in the body."*

The Englishman realized that a person who had this disorder had tremors or commonly called "shaky Palsy." It was noted that it was an incurable disease that affected the body's central nervous system.

Parkinson Disease term was coined I 1865 by William Sanders then later A French neurologist by the name of Jean-Martin was noted as the one who popularized the term.

Parkinson Disease Explained

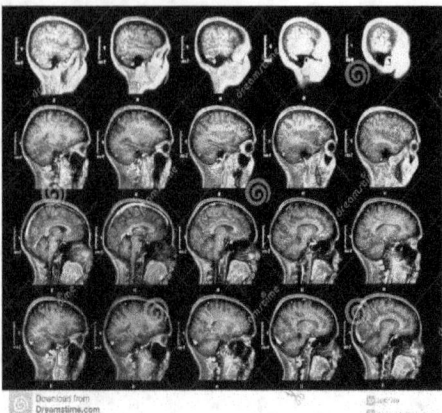

 The brain should manufacture dopamine which is a neurotransmitter but lacked the ability to do this which caused the tremors and the body to shake. Today through the Michael J Fox foundation it was discovered that many factors come into play that affect those who suffer from Parkinson.

The clinical definition declares that a person who has PD suffers from blurred vision, muscles become ridged, shuffling of the feet with a slow gait. Also, a slow slurred speech and a masked facial expression.

Many of us who have Parkinson will tell you that there are many other things that we suffer. One of the other main symptoms is called Sun Downing, nerves, lack of ability to feel in place with family and friends. Our immune system is not always good causing to get frequent bouts of flu and/or pneumonia. In ability to retain thoughts is another problem we often suffer.

Parkinson's Other Disorders

Let us look at Parkinson in a whole new light. The disease has its own problems in and of itself. However, there are other disorders that effect people with Parkinson that complicate our ability to function.

1) Sun-downing is one of the major things that affects me. Many who have PD have this problem. It is the inability to not get sleep. I have gone to date as high as four nights and days without closing my eyes. This causes me to be loopy like someone who is drinking.
2) Restless legs while many people suffer from this those of us who have PD suffer greatly. If we can get any rest this problem hinders us.
3) Dementia a problem that many seniors suffer affects PD patients.
4) Hallucinations is another problem that affects PD patients and this can stem from the medication.
5) Memory Impairment happens when certain drugs are administered to combat PD.
6) Irritable bowel may happen when anticholinergic drugs are used.
7) Anxiety drugs are often administered for those who get overly anxious. These drugs will cause PD patients to suffer from memory loss or confusion.
8) Cramps, Sciatica, Pain and Tingling is a major problem for many who suffer from PD.
9) Shortness of breath known as Dyspnea is due from PD.
10) Orthostatic Hypotension in other words some PD patients suffer from Imbalance, Vertigo, and/or Faintness because of low blood pressure.

These are just some of the many things that Parkinson Disease people suffer from and we will be discussing later in the book.

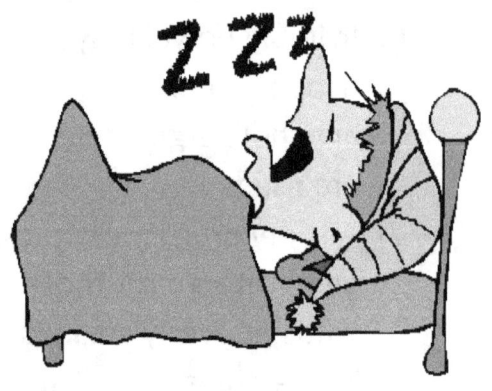

Catching Z's is not easy with Parkinson Disease

Sleep Disorders

Parkinson Disease hosts several different types of sleep disorders. One of the most common sleep disorder for those who suffer from PD is called Sun downing. Those who suffer from Sun downing find that it is caused by insufficient treatment of PD which causes the patient not to be able to get proper rest during the night. A lack of amino acid created by the brain contributes to this problem. Insomnia due to PD can last for several nights making the PD patient constantly tired.

Parkinson limits your movements in bed which prevents normal nocturnal movements. Being stuck amongst the covers makes it impossible to move while sleeping.

Akathisia of Parkinson

This is a very important factor that people with PD must overcome. This is an inner restlessness which causes you to be faced with the inability to relax. The PD person should develop habits that will help them to relax. This is necessary to overcome restlessness.

I find that it is impossible at times no matter what I do to relax so I just go with the flow. Like taking walks for instance if my legs are too restless. I have a stationary bike that I sometimes use when it is impossible for me to go outside.

Akathisia is the inner feeling of restlessness. A PD person is unable to feel relaxed a nondescript discomfort felt when sitting or lying down. Many people with PD do not reveal this to the doctors but when ask they recognize the symptoms. These symptoms are treatable. The PD patient will find that sleep problems can be handled when faced appropriately.

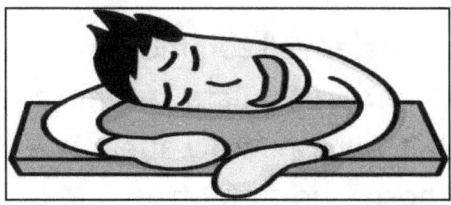

Many people like to do crafts, read books, or play games. I enjoy writing most of all. The fact remains that with PD it might boil down to an inadequate amount of Levodopa. A PD patient falls to sleep and wakes up in about two hours. The need to have the brain make enough dopamine to sleep wains when the levodopa wears out. That is why a time released dose is very helpful.

Sun downing

This is a term used for those with Parkinson Disease who are unable to get to sleep of an evening. Often when the sun goes down the PD person becomes wide awake. The fact is that most Parkinson Disease patients have their own sleep problems. It is wise to check what is happening in your life to conquer insomnia.

One wife complained that her husband would get up take his medication and then go to sleep for half the day. Then he wakes do lunch and sleep the rest of the day. It turned out that he was not taking medications after dinner so at night he was not sleepy. A change in medication schedule help cure his Sun downing problem.

Others have complained that worry about finances, family, or work have caused them to not be able to go to sleep. The brain races with many thoughts depriving the PD patient the ability to go to sleep. When this happens, it is best to consult your neurologist for sleep aids. Some PD patients find that a nice glass of wine helps relax them instead of a sleep aid.

Insomnia because of PD

Parkinson Disease people often are not able to get a good night's sleep because of the dopamine-deficient state. It is impossible to get relaxed and comfortable enough to get into a sleep-induced state. There are those who suffer with tremors, restless legs, and/or fidgety all prevent good sleep.

Not all of us suffer from the same symptoms that is why it hard to give an overall remedy for insomnia. The fact many of us have a lack of mobility makes it hard to turn or move during normal sleep. This prevents a person from getting normal sleep.

Dementia, Memory Loss, and Hallucinations

These are all common disorders that affect seniors but will especially affect those who suffer from Parkinson Disease. Normally it does not come into play until a person with PD is older or has had PD for an extended period.

Dementia comes about because of lack of dopamine in the brain. Unfortunately, the medication does not always work as our body gets use to it then we become immune. We cannot focus as well as we use to causing us to have memory loss.

Memory loss comes about because as we get older the cells in our brain do not function as good as possible. When you have PD then the dopamine is not being produced like it should and the medication is not working as well.

We find that at first, we forget simple things like where did we put our cell phone. We may discover that we are unable to remember a favorite recipe that we had made for years. But we can recall important things in our lives like who we are ha, ha.

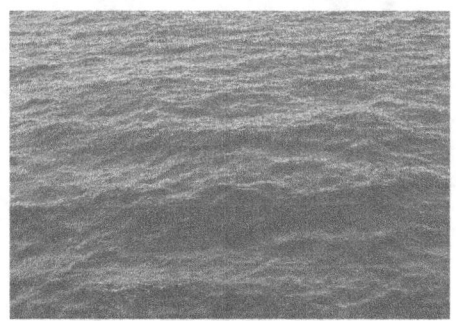

Think of calming waters

It is often necessary to have a medicine change or adjustment in the amount of PD medicine we are taking. It helps to think of things like calming waters to help relieve stress and help the sleep pattern as well as adequate amounts of medication.

Hallucinations happen to PK patients a lot of times because of the medications that need to be taken when you have Parkinson. For instance, your body might become immune to your meds so the doctor will prescribe new meds that could cause a person to hallucinate. Often the fact a person is suffering from dementia will cause them to hallucinate while on their PK meds. This is something that can be controlled by the amount of medications a person is taking.

Whether you are suffering from memory loss, dementia, or other memory problems it is essential when you hallucinate to contact your doctor immediately.

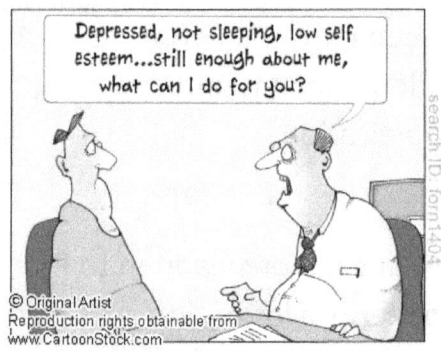

Seek Psychiatric Help When Depressed

Parkinson Disease and Psychiatrists

The fact is when you do suffer from Parkinson Disease there are times in your life when you find that you are overly depressed or just have too many worries.

This is a major problem that is hard to face by yourself because remember your brain is being attacked! Your brain lacks the substance it needs to help you overcome many of your problems. This does not mean by any means you have a mental disorder.

Simply put you need medications to help your brain manufacture the dopamine necessary to help you. In some cases, just facing the fact you have Parkinson can be overwhelming. Medications like Ativan are very helpful. Then having someone to talk to like a Psychiatrists or Psychologist is beneficial.

Suicide is not common occurrence amongst those with PD but left unchecked without proper medical help for depression it is partly possible. Your doctor is better able to prescribe medicine for you to prevent those thoughts and to help you work out problems that may cause you to have suicidal thoughts.

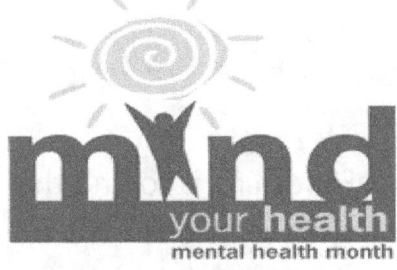

Your Worth is Found in God

Not in Opinions of Others

Parkinson Disease Depression Reasons

There are multiple reasons for a person to get depressed and in Parkinson Disease it happens to many people who suffer from the disorder. In some cases, it is the reaction to the news that a person has been diagnosed with the disease. The idea of this disability is overwhelming. Treatment of Parkinsonism shows improvement and helps a PD patient to get over the depression.

The deficiency of dopamine in the brain is a major cause of depression for a PD Patient. It is highly noticeable for people when they have a fluctuating motor response. Proper treatment helps this motor response problem and helps the PD patient regain control.

Serotonin helps when a deficiency in the brain occurs. This is caused by the neurogenerative process in the brain effects a person. This is treated by the drug Serotonin SSRI which helps a person with Parkinson Disease.

There are other brain chemistry problems that are linked to the person who suffers from Parkinson Disease. A deficiency in neurotransmitters is the cause of many problems so antidepressant drugs are used to counter the problem and help the patient with depression.

Pseudo-dementia

People who suffer from Parkinson that show signs of Pseudo-dementia may seem dull and very uninterested in any activities. Doctors evaluate these symptoms because it is treatable. Once depression is controlled in these cases then memory flow returns.

Treatments for Depression

Since there are different reasons a person might get depression with Parkinson Disease it is only safe to assume that there are multiple ways to treat depression.

Treatment strategies depend on the severity of the depression first. Then next it depends on the cause for the depression along with how the family support system.

Treatment of Depression Elements

- First thing is to find the symptoms evaluate them and determine how severe the depression is for the patient.
- Insomnia is noted as a sure sign of depression. When insomnia is noted then often levodopa therapy is used at bedtime.
- The Parkinson patient needs to try to become active. Activity is very important. Don't just sit back and keep your mind on television it only aggravates the depression.

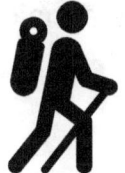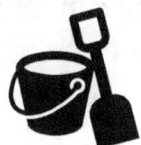

Outdoor Activities Great Way to Overcome Depression

While medications are a valuable tool to help you overcome depression it is essential that you also use other resources that are available to you.

It is very easy to sit and just watch television. But that does not solve your problems. Try activities such as taking walks, swimming, hiking, or playing games. Many people like to play baseball for instance.

Then it is possible that you like to read, do crafts, go to shopping malls, antiquing, or other forms of being active that you enjoy but have long since stopped.

Depression is a problem but it is one that can be cured if the right methods are used. See your doctor for the right medications, eat right, exercise, and get active. Be with your friends and family they are very helpful when it comes to solving your problem with depression.

Talk therapy is an excellent way to overcome depression.

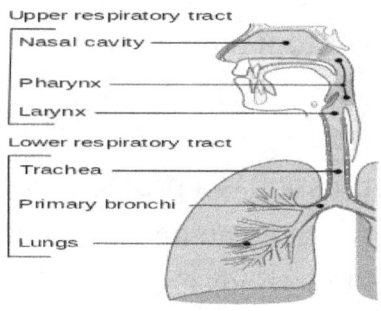

Upper respiratory tract
Nasal cavity
Pharynx
Larynx
Lower respiratory tract
Trachea
Primary bronchi
Lungs

Throat-

Choking can become a major problem.

Most patients with this problem develop pneumonia which is infection that develops in the lung. Patients who develop this problem are carefully watched by their physician. Since it is a Parkinson person who has this disorder then the same drugs are used to treat it.

A slowness in the body prevents a person from swallowing properly. The use of carbidopa/levodopa helps the Parkinson person overcome the Dysphagia problem.

Dysphagia (Swallowing)

When a person has difficult in swallowing it is referred to as Dysphagia. This is a rare problem in the start of Parkinson Disease but can develop later in the disorder.

Food and liquid pool in the mouth making it difficult for the patient to swallow.

Methods to Prevent Dysphagia

It Is helpful to do some of the following steps to help control the Dysphagia problem of swallowing.

1. When a person is eating or drinking they should sit up straight not slouch or be in a laying position.
2. Keep your chin down when trying to swallow. This helps the food to go down the right pipe.
3. It is important not to take large bites or huge gulps. Especially when eating foods like meat because they can get stuck in your throat very easily.
4. Do not eat at a fast pace slow down and chew your foods properly.
5. When you find that solid foods are a problem then wash them down with liquids. Water is the best liquid to use.
6. When the problem becomes overwhelming then use foods that are easy enough for you swallow. You can eat purred foods, puddings, and creamed dishes.
7. Experiment with liquids see if ice cold liquids are easier to manage with your foods or do you need warmer liquids.
8. When you find water and soda seem to go down the wrong pipe choking you then try things like milkshakes. You can add a thickener to your liquids if needed to help you in swallowing.

Finally, if swallowing becomes a major problem then you should consult a swallowing expert. There are doctors who focus on this problem who can help. Dysphagia is a major problem that can be handled to prevent any diet deficiency

The simple Foods Can become a problem to eat

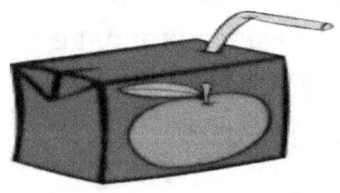

Other methods can be used to still be able to enjoy foods.

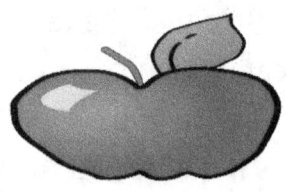

Speech and Voice

In some cases, speech is affected making it very difficult to pronounce certain sounds. Articulation soon becomes a problem as you advance in the PD. Some people may claim that they cannot hear you but that is because you are speaking to softly.

It is even more difficult for seniors because hearing loss makes them understand you even less. The first thing that should be done is the optimizing of your medication. Speaking takes using muscles just like walking.

Losing the ability to express yourself is very frustrating. Many people who start to have this problem become depressed. Often, they find that the ability to eat is also a problem and drooling often happens as well.

These things are usually handled by adjustments to the PD patient's medications. Often a person who suffers from PD finds that it is time to increase the Carbidopa/Levodopa intake.

Medications Overviews

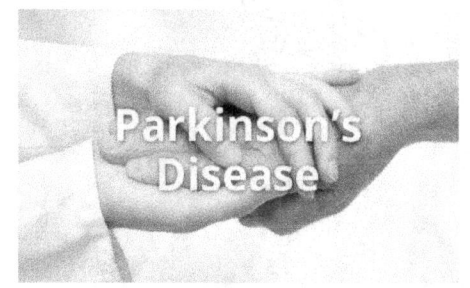

Touch A Hand Make a Friend

1. **Apokyn**- is a prescription drug approved by the Food and Drug Administration (FDA) in 2004 to treat intermittent "off" episode in people with advanced Parkinson's Disease.

   Apomorphine is the drugs name. A drug referred to as an antiemetic may be given to prevent nausea and vomiting. Trimethobenzamide is often taken along with the Apomorphine.

   This drug is in the dopamine family imitating the action needed of dopamine in the brain. Often prescribed for those in the advanced stages of Parkinson Disease.

Medication Overview Continued

2. Overview
   Artane is a prescription drug approved by the Food and Drug Administration (FDA) in 1949 to treat motor symptoms in all forms of Parkinsonism. Artane is often prescribed to younger people with Parkinson's Disease. Artane is also referred to by its drug name, trihexyphenidyl.

   Artane is not suitable for use in people with tardive dyskinesia or narrow-angle glaucoma, or who have previously shown hypersensitivity to trihexyphenidyl. Artane must be used with caution in people with mental disorders, arteriosclerosis, enlarged prostate, fast heart rate (tachycardia), liver or kidney disease, or problems with the heart, stomach, or blood pressure. Artane may not be appropriate...

3. **Overview**

   Azilect is a prescription drug approved by the Food and Drug Administration (FDA) in 2006 to treat motor symptoms in people with Parkinson's Disease. **Azilect** may be prescribed as a monotherapy to people with early Parkinson's Disease, or as an adjunctive (add-on) treatment in those who are taking **Levodopa/Carbidopa** and experiencing reductions in its effectiveness. **Azilect** is also referred to by its drug name, **rasagiline.**

   Azilect is not suitable for use in people with a major psychotic disorder or those who have previously

shown hypersensitivity to rasagiline. Azilect must be used with caution in people with high blood pressure, mental illness, or liver or kidney problem

4. **Overview**

   Cogentin is a prescription drug approved by the Food and Drug Administration (FDA) in 1954 to treat motor symptoms in all forms of Parkinsonism. Cogentin is often prescribed to younger people with Parkinson's Disease. Cogentin is also referred to by its drug name, Benztropine mesylate.

   Cogentin is not suitable for use in people with tardive dyskinesia or angle-closure glaucoma, or who have previously shown hypersensitivity to Benztropine mesylate. Cogentin must be used with caution in people with mental disorders, enlarged prostate, fast heart rate (tachycardia), liver or kidney disease, or problems with the heart, stomach, or blood pressure. Cogentin may not be appropriate for women who are pregnant or breastfeeding.

Cogentin is a member of a class of drugs called anticholinergics. Cogentin is believed to work by influencing the balance of brain chemicals called neurotransmitters. Neurotransmitters enable the transmission of messages between nerves.

5. Overview
   Cotman is a prescription drug approved by the Food and Drug Administration (FDA) in 1999. Cotman is prescribed as an adjunct (add-on) drug to Levodopa/Carbidopa if the latter drugs begin to lose effectiveness in treating motor symptoms of Parkinson's Disease. Combined with Levodopa/Carbidopa, Cotman may provide some benefit for those with Progressive Supranuclear Palsy, Vascular Parkinsonism, Multiple System **Atrophy,** and **Corticobasa**l Degeneration. Cotman is also known by its drug name, nitecapone.

Cotman is not appropriate for people with a major psychotic disorder or a history of hypersensitivity to entacapone. **Cotman** must be used with caution in people with hypotension, colitis, mental illness, alcoholism, or problems with the heart, kidneys, liver, lungs, or blood vessels. Cotman may not be appropriate for women who are pregnant or breastfeeding.

6. Overview
   Duopa is a prescription drug approved by the Food and Drug Administration (FDA) in 2015 to treat fluctuating motor symptoms in those with advanced Parkinson's Disease. **Duopa** may be prescribed if your condition is responsive to dopaminergic treatment, but you have three or more hours of "off" time on your current drug regimen.

Duopa is not appropriate for people with undiagnosed skin lesions, narrow-angle glaucoma, or a history of melanoma, stomach ulcers, or stomach surgery.

Duopa is not suitable for use in people who have previously shown hypersensitivity to Levodopa or Carbidopa. **Duopa** must be used with caution in people with wide-angle glaucoma, diabetes, asthma, emphysema, mental illness, or problems with the heart, kidneys, liver, lungs, or blood vessels. **Duopa** may not be appropriate for women who are pregnant or breastfeeding.

Duopa is a combination drug containing both **Levodopa and Carbidopa**. Levodopa is the precursor molecule to the neurotransmitter Dopamine. Levodopa is believed to treat Parkinsonian motor symptoms by increasing the concentration of Dopamine in the brain.

Carbidopa is a molecule that inhibits the breakdown of **Levodopa** into **Dopamine** before it reaches the brain. Carbidopa is believed to work by increasing the amount of Levodopa that reaches the brain, making Levodopa effective at significantly lower doses.

Generic Drugs

Some medications are available both as generic and branded products. Although generic and branded formulations of a drug contain the same active ingredients at the same concentrations, your body may react differently to different formulations. Check with your doctor before switching between drug brands or between generic and branded drugs.

Deep Brain Stimulation

Overview
People with Parkinson's Disease whose motor symptoms are debilitating and cannot be controlled with medications, or whose side effects from medications are severe, may be candidates for Deep Brain Stimulation (DBS). Candidates must have intact cognitive function and be healthy enough to undergo three to six hours of surgery while awake.

While DBS can relieve motor symptoms of Parkinson's Disease, it is not a cure for Parkinson's Disease.

What does it involve?

Your neurologist will perform extensive testing to find out whether you are a good candidate for DBS. The pre-surgical evaluation tests may include magnetic resonance imaging (MRI) scans and computed tomography (CT) scans. Pre-surgical evaluation is very thorough to ensure you will receive the maximum possible benefit from the surgery and avoid disruptions of normal brain function.

You and your doctor should decide together whether DBS may be right for you. Do not be afraid to ask questions about any aspect of the surgery or recovery.

DBS involves the implantation of a three-part device to block electrical signals that cause tremors and other motor symptoms of Parkinson's.

DBS is implanted in two different surgeries. The first surgery is usually performed while you are awake, with a local anesthetic to numb your scalp.

Your head will be kept perfectly still by a device called a stereotactic frame. Remaining conscious will allow you to answer the surgeon's questions and help them pinpoint the correct locations for the electrodes.

The surgeon will place a fine wire and four small electrodes into your brain, and a small generator device (also called the neurostimulator) will be placed near your collarbone.

A thin wire will be inserted under your skin to connect the electrodes with the neurostimulator. The first

27

surgery will take three to six hours. You can expect to stay in the hospital for two to three days after this surgery.

The second surgery will happen about a week later. You will be under general anesthetic for this surgery, which will involve placing a pulse generator device containing batteries on your chest wall. The surgeon will also insert a small wire under your skin connecting the pulse generator and the neurostimulator. You will likely spend less than 24 hours in the hospital after the second surgery. A doctor or nurse will educate you on how to care for your wounds.

You will need to take antibiotics to prevent infection while you are recovering at home from the surgeries. You may feel tired, and the surgical sites may be sore.

Avoid even light activity such as sex or cleaning the house for the first two weeks. Do not perform heavier activities such as exercise or most types of work for four to six weeks after surgery.

After a few weeks, you will visit your neurologist's office to program and activate your DBS system. The neurologist controls the amount and frequency of stimulation, and you can turn the device on and off with a magnetic remote control.

You will need to stay in close communication with your neurologist to ensure that your DBS is functioning optimally. The battery for your DBS should last three to five years.

Exercise

Exercise can help everyone stay healthy and feel their best. For people with Parkinson's, exercise offers important additional benefits.

Getting regular exercise can reduce motor symptoms of Parkinson's, slow the progression of the disease, and improve mood. A regular exercise routine can also help protect against the development of Parkinson's in those who may be at risk.

Why Exercise

Always check with your doctor before beginning a new exercise regimen. Consider consulting with a physical therapist to develop a customized exercise plan. Most types of exercise can be adapted to accommodate those with Parkinson's.

People with any stage or severity of Parkinson's Disease can benefit from exercise. Doctors and researchers agree that the more exercise you do, the more benefit you will receive from the activity. Research also indicates that the more intensely you exercise, the better. When you exercise, do it intensely enough that your heart beats faster and you are breathing hard.

Whatever type of exercise you choose, follow these general safety guidelines. Always begin your workout session with a gradual warm-up and take time to cool down afterward. Warming up and cooling down will help prevent sore or pulled muscles. Exercise should be somewhat challenging, but never a struggle. Stay hydrated with plenty of cool liquids, choosing beverages without caffeine.

It is important to choose a type of exercise you will enjoy. Consider joining a dance class, boxing class, or yoga class to keep you motivated and incorporate social aspects. Aerobic exercise can take many forms.

Walking on a treadmill, riding a stationary or recumbent bike, climbing stairs, or swimming can all provide effective exercise. Resistance training such as lifting weights can be done seated, and it can involve as light a weight as you are comfortable lifting.

Even small amounts of weight or resistance – for instance, lifting your arms or legs repeatedly against gravity – provide benefits. Be creative. Activities such as gardening and walking a pet can help you stay active and healthy.

It is important not to become discouraged early on when beginning an exercise regimen. At first, try to exercise for 10 minutes each day. As you become accustomed to the activity, exercise for longer periods every day. Focus on finding ways of staying active that are safe, enjoyable and easy to do regularly. If you experience new or worse

Parkinson's symptoms or side effects from medications, adjust your workout program to keep it safe and rewarding.

Regular, intense exercise has also been proven to help protect against the development of Parkinson's Disease.

Some neurologists recommend that people who have relatives with Parkinson's maintain a rigorous exercise routine to decrease their risk.

Intended Outcomes

Exercise can help you achieve and maintain your best physical and psychological condition. A regular exercise regimen can reduce Parkinson's symptoms such as tremor, gait, coordination, flexibility, and grip strength. Exercise might protect your brain from disease progression. Regular exercise can help you avoid falls and recover more quickly. Physical exercise can increase strength, promote healthy weight, stave off heart disease and osteoporosis, and improve your mood and self-esteem.

Results of Exercise

An article published in 2014 studied exercise in 4,866 people with Parkinson's Disease. After one year, participants who exercised regularly showed better quality of life, less cognitive decline, improved mobility, function, and mood, and less burden for caregivers.

Diet for Better Health

Many of us eat while on the run because of our busy schedule. This is not advisable for those with Parkinson Disease.

We need to be ever mindful of what we eat and how much we eat. PD people should consult their doctor when it comes to losing weight or gaining weight. Being overweight can cause other health issues.

It is essential to realize that being underweight is also a health risk.

You need to formulate a diet plan that is suitable to your needs. I myself was over-weight become a diabetic and found other health problems arising.

I had visited my doctor about my obesity with no luck. I had tried diet programs no luck. Then one day I decided to sit down and put together a good diet and exercise program for myself. I knew good foods from the bad ones and what would not interfere with my medications.

My Diet Plan

This was the diet plan I put together myself and within three months I went from 210 lbs. to 150 lbs. I felt that I knew what my body needed and understood the concepts of a good diet that is why I made up a diet plan that was healthy for me.

Breakfast

I drink one Vanilla Protein Shake every morning. Since I am so hooked on caffeine I drink Kellogg's Vanilla Cappuccino. Then I go and ride the bicycle now for half an hour and drink a bottle of water while I am doing this.

Lunches

My lunches are very easy to do and very healthy as well. I eat things like cheese and crackers, cold meats, fresh fruits like watermelon, peanut butter, all the good things for you.

Dinner

At this point I usually eat a good wholesome meal but not over eat.

I eat a lot of chicken and fish! Some beef but not often. Pork can be eaten but it depends on what and how you fix it.

I like my rice and pasta! But know it is not good to have a lot every week. I like to make fresh garden salad using lettuce, tomatoes, cucumber some carrots, celery, hard-boiled egg with some ham or turkey mixed into the salad.

A good pasta dish occasionally but just doesn't over eat. Baked chicken is for my Sunday dinner along with mashed potatoes and corn on the cob.

All my meals are prepared for me by me not the box mixes. I do like to use the slow cooker it helps to cut back on oil intake and helps flavor up the foods. There are many things you can do for yourself when you think about your diet plan.

Foods to Avoid with PARKINSON'S DISEASE

The medication <u>levodopa</u> (Sinemet) is a protein building block so it competes for absorption with other proteins. Eating a very proteinic meal reduces the likelihood of effectively absorbing levodopa, so you may want to leave meat, fish and cheese for dinner and eat more carbohydrates and vegetables during the day.

Taking medication on an empty stomach -- 30 minutes before or 60 minutes after a meal -- allows the drug to reach the small intestine and absorb faster.

However, a carbohydrate snack (crackers, toast, oatmeal) with the medication may be necessary to prevent nausea.

Dopamine agonists (pramipexole and ropinirole) do not require any dietetic adjustment. Those who take MAO-B inhibitors (rasagiline or selegiline) should eat with moderation -- but not eliminate -- foods that contain high concentrations of tyramine. MAO-B

inhibitors increase tyramine, and the combination could elevate blood pressure. This list of foods to avoid includes:

- cured, fermented or air-dried meats or fish
- aged cheeses: aged cheddar or Swiss, blue cheeses, Camembert
- fermented cabbage: sauerkraut, kimchi
- soybean products, including soy sauce
- red wine and tap beer
  Iron supplements can also decrease absorption of levodopa so they should be separated from medications by at least two hours.

DIETARY CHANGES CAN EASE PARKINSON'S SYMPTOMS?

Constipation is common in Parkinson's disease. Increased fluid and fiber consumption can help maintain regularity. Aim to drink six to eight 8-ounce glasses of water per day.

Warm liquids, especially in the morning, can stimulate bowel movements. Dietary sources of fiber consist of fruits (with the peel), vegetables, legumes, whole grain breads and cereals.

Most of these are high in antioxidants as well.
Low blood pressure is a symptom of Parkinson's and a side effect of some medications. Raising fluid and salt intake will boost blood pressure, but talk with your physician, especially if you have heart or kidney problems. Increase cold fluids -- water, Gatorade, V8 juice -- to five 8-ounce glasses per half day.

Limit caffeinated beverages, hot liquids and alcohol as these encourage dehydration and low blood pressure. Eating frequent, small meals can also smooth blood pressure fluctuations.

Swallowing problems can present as coughing, choking or a sensation of food feeling "stuck."

A speech therapist can prescribe appropriate, individualized dietary modifications and adaptive strategies. These may include adding foods with increased "sensory input" (e.g., seasoned, cold, sour or carbonated items) or altering the consistency of solids and/or liquids. In addition, you might be asked to sit up straight, take smaller bites at a slower pace and allow for longer mealtimes.

Some people with Parkinson's experience painful muscle cramping, especially at night and as medication wears off. Eating yellow mustard, which contains the spice turmeric, or drinking tonic water, which contains quinine, may help. Others endorse salt, vinegar or pickle juice. Maintaining adequate hydration may prevent or limit cramping.

ANTIOXIDANTS AND WHAT FOODS CONTAIN THEM?

Antioxidants are one of those "good for you" things you hear about all the time. They're molecules that clear out free radicals -- toxic substances formed from stresses like air pollution, sunlight, cigarette smoke and even the process of converting food to energy. Oxidative stress is a biological condition caused by too many free radicals. It's associated with aging and Parkinson's disease, so a diet high in antioxidants may offset oxidative stress and cellular damage.

Antioxidants in Foods:

- vegetables: artichokes, okra, kale, bell peppers, potatoes
- fruits: berries, pears, apples, grapes
- grains
- eggs
- legumes: kidney beans, edamame, lentils
- nuts: pecans, walnuts, hazelnuts
- dark chocolate
- some beverages such as red wine, coffee and tea

SHOULD I EAT FAVA BEANS OR ANY OTHER SPECIFIC FOODS?

Fava beans contain levodopa, so adding them to one's diet is an attractive idea. Unfortunately, the concentration and availability of levodopa in fava beans are unknown and likely minimal. No other special foods are recommended for those with Parkinson's disease. Talk to your doctor or dietitian to craft a diet **that helps you manage your Parkinson's symptoms and feel energized and healthy.**

* NOTE: The medical information contained in this article is for general information purposes only. It is crucial that care and treatment decisions related to Parkinson's disease and any other medical condition be made in consultation with a physician or other qualified medical professional. While some of the information comes from the Michael J Fox

Other Problems for PD Patients Suffered

While a person with Parkinson Disease suffers greatly from the disease itself as you can see other problems do occur. Many times, those other problems can be just as devastating as Parkinson itself.

Drooling & Swallowing

Lack of the right medication or not enough medication can result in a PD patient having problems with drooling and swallowing. This can be resolved by a medication adjustment. Botulinum Toxin injections are used for those with serious problem.

Speech and Voice Problems

Problems arise for PD patients at times because of their inability to speak properly. The voice may get very low and shallow. This is treated by medication adjustments plus speech therapy.

Digestive Problems & Constipation Problems

Many times, PD patients find that they have digestive problems that could result in constipation because they are not able to chew their food properly.

There is a valve between the stomach and lower intestine that effects the PD patient.

There is a delay in stomach emptying which causes bloating and at times nausea. All this adds up to digestive problems and constipation.

The Parkinson Body

It is inevitable that those who suffer from PD also have multiple things go wrong with their body. They suffer from their internal organs having problems. The urinary tract, bowels, kidneys, lungs, breathing, headaches, sleep deprivation, swelling of the feet and legs, and heart problems. All these problems can be taken care of if properly handled with the right medications.

Life vs Death

Life for a Parkinson person can be fruitful if they wish to make it that way. Many activities can be done. The family can be enjoyed, vacations done, jobs can be maintained life in general can be maintained. It is up to the person who suffers from PK to take control of their life.

How we live and the quality of life we have can be awesome if we only take care of ourselves. There are many avenues we can use to gain better health and longer lasting life. People with Parkinson Disease will live a very long life if they maintain a good diet, exercise and take the right medications.

Depression and other emotional problems often attack Parkinson people but with therapy it can all be worked out. Your fate in other words is in your own hands.

Your belief in God will help you get through those rough times. Family and friends are essential as well to help you overcome and pursue a very good life.

Family Togetherness

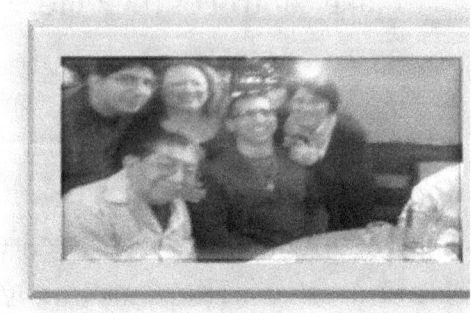

My Life

While my life has not always been easy I do not have complaints. It took me some time to get settled into an existence that I could accept.

Parkinson Disease can be devastating if you let it. Everything in our lives can become a catastrophe or it can be a new challenge.

It is up to each person how they handle cope with life's problems. Parkinson Disease is not my only problems I have had many over the years. Diagnosed with polio when 35 years old in my left side, head trauma from an auto accident, difficult pregnancy, and all my immediately family has long since died. So, you see life is not an easy thing but death?

I have learned to take each thing at the time and with my faith in God I have overcome. Why these things happen? It is my life's highway of challenge.

I want to encourage each one of you to be brave take that one step forward and face the day with a smile.

Find your niche in life. What makes you happy? Don't worry about tomorrow. Live today with gusto and a smile!

It does not matter if you have Parkinson Disease or some

other ailment if you have life then live it.

Take the challenge! Be not afraid! God is with you always!

Author----Shirley J. Lopez

IBN#